# THE ULTIMATE KETO MEAL PREP GUIDE

## A Complete Guide to Easy Meal Prep

# Table of Contents

# Introduction

The Ultimate Keto Meal Prep Guide is the perfect introduction to understanding the Ketogenic diet and learning about easy keto meal prep.

This guide explains, in simple terms, the science behind how the ketogenic diet works. It tells you, which foods you can and cannot eat, and gives you a range of tasty food options that will keep you satisfied.

The keto diet is ideal for those who want to lose weight quickly, without the associated hunger experiences with most other diets.

By following the Keto diet, you will:

- Convert body fat into sustainable energy
- Stabilize your body's insulin and blood sugar levels
- Lower high blood pressure and reduce bad cholesterol
- Give you more energy
- Help you to think more clearly

A ketogenic diet is a high fat, moderate protein, low carbohydrate way of eating. It dispels the myths of other diets that eating fat is bad. With the keto diet, sugar in all its forms is the enemy. But rather than eating bland food in tiny portions, on the keto diet, you can eat lots of delicious, filling foods that will keep you satisfied and still let you lose weight. Read on to find out more.

# Chapter 1: Why Choose a Ketogenic Diet

The Ketogenic diet has been around for a while now, but rather than be a short-lived fad, it has endured. In this ultimate keto meal prep guide, we will teach you the science behind the ketogenic diet and share with you delicious easy to prepare meals that will keep you satisfied.

The ketogenic diet works by burning fat instead of glucose. Glucose is the body's "go to" energy source, but by using ketogenic principles you teach your body to stop using glucose and instead to use fat to supply you with energy. There are many advantages to this, so let's look at some of them:

- **Lowers cholesterol and blood pressure** – many people have high cholesterol, which can be problematic to health. By using a ketogenic diet, you can retrain your body to use fat instead of glucose as its main energy source. Most of this fat comes from your own fat stores. This isn't something that happens overnight but can take a while to achieve. As your body becomes used to using fat for energy instead of glucose your blood cholesterol will decrease along with your blood pressure.
- **Cravings** – On a keto diet you can eat a lot more foods with high fat content and this stops hunger cravings from happening. When the body is using fat for energy, the energy is released far more slowly and in a more balanced way than when your body is using glucose for energy. This means you don't have energy highs and lows and your body doesn't think you are about to enter a starvation phase and demand you eat 3 bowls of cereal (for example).
- **Insulin release** – No doubt you have heard about insulin and recognize it as being a factor in diabetes. Insulin is responsible for telling the cells in your body that they need to take up the glucose and use it for energy. Glucose is made in the body as our primary energy source and it is converted from sugar and carbohydrate that we eat. If glucose spikes insulin levels in the body and if they continue to be spiked the body's cells stop listening to the insulin messages telling them to use the glucose, so the body then releases even more insulin. This is known as insulin resistance and is a precursor for diabetes.

  If you are a diabetic the ketogenic diet can help you to regain control of your blood sugar levels.

- **Epilepsy** – Interestingly it has been noted that children with epilepsy who eat a ketogenic diet have fewer seizures. Why this should be so is not yet fully understood, but research is ongoing.
- **Weight loss** - If you are searching for a good weight loss method that gets rid of your fat, then the ketogenic diet is a perfect solution. In order to

burn fat, your body needs to have no available glucose to use, as it will always use glucose for energy before fat (essentially because it is easier to do) and excess glucose is then turned into fat. To make the body use fat for energy, you need to take it to a stage called ketosis. This requires stopping your intake of foods that convert to glucose and eating foods that are high in fat instead.  The ketones produced when your body is in ketosis, ensure that your brain is supplied with enough energy too.

# Chapter 2: How Using the Ketogenic Diet Works

It sounds great, using a diet that uses our fat stores instead of glucose, that if left unused just turns to fat. But, making the body achieve this fat burning state takes a bit of understanding.

By replacing almost all the carbohydrates and all the refined sugar that you currently consume and replacing it with healthy fats, your body will enter a state called ketosis, which is what gives the Ketogenic or Keto diet its name.

When you are using a ketogenic diet, you need to keep a balanced macronutrient ratio. This is the percentage of fat you consume against the amount of protein and carbohydrate. A good macronutrient balance for a standard keto diet would look something like this:

- Fat 60% to 80%
- Protein 15% to 35%
- Carbohydrate 5% or less

To help you with this it is a good idea to use a keto macro calculator. These can be found online and will calculate the best ratio for your body's requirements.

If you stick to the macronutrient ratios your body will, after a few days, enter the state called ketosis, where it uses ketones for energy instead of glucose.

Ketones are produces when your body starts to break down fat that it needs to use for energy. Ketones are made in the liver when the body no longer has enough glucose (called glycogen when being used in the body) to provide energy. The process in the liver is called beta-oxidation and is how ketones are formed to be used for fuel.

We produce three different types of ketones in the body, these are:

- Acetoacetate
- Beta-hydroxybutyric acid (not strictly a ketone but used in the process)
- Acetone

The ketones that transport energy from our liver to the body's cells are Acetoacetate and beta-hydroxybutyric acid. The acetoacetate is formed by breaking down fatty acids, which are converted into either beta-hydroxybutyric acid or acetone. Acetone is not a useful ketone for energy and is simply expelled in the breath. This gives someone who is in ketosis the typical acetone breath odor and it smells rather like pear drops.

Because the body is programmed to always use glucose rather than fat for energy, our modern carbohydrate rich diet is causing big problems. Obesity and diet related diseases such as diabetes, cancer and heart problems are increasing at alarming levels. This was not such a problem for our ancestors as their diet would typically have contained far fewer simple starchy carbs and sugars such as fructose syrup and corn syrup would not have been an added ingredient to almost everything. This is a sad reflection on our lazy ways as we often prefer to buy readymade food products that are filled with many ingredients that are not so good for our health, rather than take the time and effort to make our own.

### *Where do the sugars come from and what do they do?*

- Glucose comes from starch carbohydrate foods that include bread, pasta, rice and potatoes. The more refined these products are, the easier it is for our body to turn them into glucose very quickly. Whole grain bread, whole wheat pasta, brown or wild rice and potatoes with their skin all slow down glucose production as the fiber content in them makes them take longer to digest. Glucose is a monosaccharide as it is one carbohydrate molecule.
- Fructose is a carbohydrate that can be found in fruit, honey and flowers, like glucose it is also a monosaccharide.
- Sucrose, which you may be more familiar with as regular table sugar is also found in fruits and vegetables. It is a disaccharide as it has two units, one fructose molecule and one glucose molecule joined together. Digestion in the body breaks them down into their two monosaccharide parts.

If you ate toast with jam for breakfast, the wheat in the toast would contain glucose as the toast is bread and therefore a carbohydrate. The jam is a combination of both fructose and sucrose, both natural and added. The body will break down the three different sugars into their individual monosaccharides. This chemical process begins in the mouth where enzymes break down the macromolecules into even smaller ones.

Once the molecules reach the stomach and enter your small intestine the pancreatic enzymes break them down still further until they are transformed into their single subunits. This allows the body to absorb them.

The small intestine has special channels that open when a sugar molecule is present. These channels then transport the sugar molecule through to your bloodstream. Once in the bloodstream, the sugar molecules are taken to the liver where they are all converted to glucose. Depending on what requirements your body has, the liver can do three things with the glucose:

- Store it as glycogen so it can be used when the body has a demand for more energy.
- Convert it to fat if there is already enough glycogen stored and the body has no immediate need for energy.
- Release the glucose through the bloodstream so it can reach parts of the body that need it for energy.

By depriving the body of enough glucose to use for energy consumption it is forced into ketosis and into using ketones. Ketones are a better source of energy for the brain, but they are not the brain's preferred source. This is because getting energy from glucose is a far easier process than having to create ketones.

As your body learns to use ketones any cravings you had will subside, your mental performance is generally also enhanced, and you will experience a better energy balance through the day. This is because using glucose for energy causes energy crashes that can make you feel tired and give you brain fog. When the body is working on ketones the energy release is a lot more stable and consistent throughout the day.

It takes the average person about two weeks to change from glucose energy production to ketone energy production. The downside of this is that you may experience withdrawal symptoms as your body is not used to having so little glucose. These symptoms will pass, and it is necessary to push through them they are sometimes called the Keto Flu and can include:

- **Brain fog** – it can be difficult to think clearly to begin with. But soon you will find your mental clarity better than it was before.
- **Digestion upset** – it is common to experience either constipation or diarrhea while your body adjusts to the fat rich diet. The symptoms will soon disappear.
- **Cold or flu symptoms** – many people feel under the weather as if they have the beginning of a cold or flu for a few days, this will soon resolve.
- **Headaches** are a very common side effect. It is important to maintain a good level of hydration, so drink plenty of water. The headaches will typically subside after a few days.
- **Sweet cravings** – it is normal to crave all foods that will supply the body with glucose. Try to maintain a steady food intake to help curb these cravings by eating fat bombs between meals. Avoid giving in to the cravings, as allowing yourself to fall victim to temptation will bring your body out of ketosis and you will have to start the process all over again.
- **Sleep disturbances** – changing your body's fuel source can cause quite a bit of disturbance on your body and this includes your hormone production when your body is getting used to running on a ketogenic diet. Sleep hormones are just one of the sets of hormones that can be affected, and it can take a week or two for your body to re-set. The best way of helping this is by consuming foods such as nuts and seeds or meat and fish.
- **Energy levels** – while your body adjusts from using glucose to using fat it will have some effect on your energy levels. Very soon you will notice an improvement and will benefit from having sustained energy throughout the day.

- **Poor mood** – carbohydrates stimulate your brains happy chemicals and while your brain becomes accustomed to not getting large hits of sugar, it will cause a disturbance in your brain's happy chemicals until it adjusts and becomes used to using ketones. To help counteract the effects try stimulating your happy chemicals in other ways. This can be done by exercising, listening to music, using soothing essential oils such as lavender or drinking herbal teas such as chamomile.
- **The wobbles** – some people have difficulty regulating their blood sugar and if this is something that happens to you, you may find you get the shakes or become light headed. This will soon pass but be careful if you are driving or operating machinery.

All these symptoms of withdrawal are normal, and they will get better. Look on them as being a good sign that your body is adjusting from using glucose to using ketones and that the addiction of sugar is being overcome. Suffering a little now will soon let you reap the rewards and you will soon no doubt begin to feel the benefits.

# How Do You Like the Book So Far?



If you're undecided, just leave a review later…

# Chapter 3: Getting Started on Keto

Before jumping right in and starting on a ketogenic diet, it is highly advisable to first talk to your doctor. This is the case whenever you decide to make a large change in your diet or fitness regime.

When you have the green light from your doctor you are best to start by getting to know yourself and the way you eat a little better. Here are some guidelines to help you:

Keep a daily food diary – By keeping a small notebook with you at all times where you can mark down EVERYTHING you eat or drink throughout the day, you can soon become familiar of any patterns. It is also advisable to note the values of the food and drink you are consuming, by checking them against an online macronutrient calculator. Don't forget to calculate the right macro balance for you as this will give you the best results.

Make a shopping list before entering the shops, this will help you to buy only the foods you need and not impulse buy high carb or high sugar food. Also make sure to clear your kitchen of any of these types of food, as this is the best way of illuminating temptation.

Although it is unlikely you will be affected by all the symptoms listed in the keto flu, you will doubtlessly suffer a few of them. Make a note of any you are experiencing in your diary, so you can see how quickly things improve and see what causes you setbacks.

There is no need to count calories on a keto diet. If you want to lose weight more rapidly, once you have allowed your body to detox and are in full ketosis (approx. 2 weeks if you don't have any setbacks), then you can also use intermittent fasting to remove the weight more rapidly. Intermittent fasting requires that you only eat in a particular time frame each day and a typical example would be only eating between the hours of 2 p.m. and 6 p.m. each day, giving you a 4-hour eating window each day.

You are on a high FAT diet, and NOT a high protein diet. Protein will stimulate insulin production and can negate the effects of a ketogenic diet as the body turns protein into glucose, so protein must be consumed in small quantities only.

It often seems very strange to be eating large quantities of fat, particularly when we have been brainwashed for so many years to believe that the only way to lose weight and improve health was by eating a low-fat diet. Do not be afraid, by eating the right kinds of fats in excess of 70% of your daily calorie intake you will be doing good! Just get used to buying full fat everything including cheese, yogurt, milk, cream, using animal fats, coconut oil and so on. It's funny how vegetables you may not particularly like, become a whole lot tastier when smothered in butter!

Fat bombs can be a total life saver if you get the munchies and need a quick fix snack. These high fat treats are easy to make and totally delicious!

### *Net Carb Counting*

When you are working out the correct macronutrient ratios for your ketogenic diet, you will need to know how to count net carbs. A net carb is the total value of carbohydrates a food contains less the fiber content. You can look up contents on the United States Department of Agriculture Food Composition Database https://ndb.nal.usda.gov/ndb/search/list the database uses grams as their unit of measurement, so 100 grams of raw broccoli is shown as having 6.64 grams of carbohydrate and 2.6 grams of dietary fiber, so the net carbohydrate is 4.06 grams. You can then easily convert the grams into ounces as necessary, by using an online converter.

Keto recipes usually have the full nutrient breakdown with all the foods macronutrient values given. It's a good idea to write them into your food diary so you can calculate what you have eaten each day.

### *Are you in Ketosis?*

When you're first starting out, it can be hard to know if you are in ketosis or not. The length of time it takes individuals to reach ketosis can differ and it can take longer when you first start. Normally, it takes anywhere between 2 and 14 days to enter ketosis. This will depend on your age, sex, body type and level of activity. Look out for the pear drops smell on your breath as an indicator that you are in ketosis. If you prefer a more scientific approach, you can also buy a special electronic device that measures ketones in your blood. These cost around $40 to $60 and you will also need to purchase the test strips to go with it. Breath tests and urine tests are also available but are not as accurate.

# Chapter 4: List of Ketogenic Foods

Here is a list of foods that are considered Ketogenic, to help you make the best choices. Avoid foods that are not listed.

### *Dairy Foods*

- Butter
- Heavy whipping cream
- Sour cream
- Full fat yogurt
- Full fat milk
- All full fat cheeses including Cheddar, parmesan, blue, brie, Colby, cottage, cream, feta, goat, Monterey Jack, mozzarella, string, swiss.

### *Meat*

- Beef: All cuts that are not lean, these include steak, roast beef, prime rib, baby back ribs, corned beef, hamburgers and so on.
- Pork: All cuts and joints (ensure you check the ingredients of processed meats as they can contain sugars).
- Lamb: All joints and cuts.

### *Poultry*

- Chicken: Breast if eaten with the skin, thighs, wings, legs, tenders and ground, whole, eggs, broth, canned (read the tin for added ingredients).
- Turkey: Breast, legs, ground.
- Duck, Goose, Pheasant, Quail: Eggs and meat.

### *Seafood*

- Fish: All oily fish including anchovies, sardines, bass, catfish, cod, flounder, haddock, halibut, herring, orange roughy, salmon, sardines, sole, tilapia, trout, tuna fish, canned salmon & tuna.
- Shellfish: (Shellfish do contain some carbs, so eat more sparingly) Crab, oysters' scallops, shrimp and other shellfish.

### *Vegetables*

- Artichokes
- Asparagus
- Avocado
- Beansprouts
- Bell peppers
- Bok choy
- Broccoli
- Brussel sprouts
- Cabbage

- Cauliflower
- Celery
- Cucumbers
- Eggplant
- Green beans
- Greens
- Hot peppers
- Kale
- Leeks
- Lettuce
- Mushrooms
- Okra
- Olives
- Onions
- Radishes
- Snow peas
- Spaghetti squash
- Spinach
- Squash
- Sweet potatoes
- Zucchini.

### *Canned Vegetables*

- Artichoke hearts
- Asparagus
- Olives
- Green beans
- Greens
- Mushrooms
- Pickles
- Sauerkraut
- Spinach

### *Fruit (Fresh)*

- Apples
- Apricots
- Avocado
- Bananas
- Blackberries
- Cherries
- Cranberries
- Figs
- Grapes (limit intake as high in sugar)
- Grapefruit
- Guava
- Kiwi

- Lemons
- Limes
- Mango
- Melons
- Nectarines
- Oranges (Clementine, Mandarin, Satsuma)
- Papaya
- Passionfruit
- Peaches
- Pears
- Pineapples
- Plums
- Pomegranates
- Raspberry
- Rhubarb
- Strawberries
- Tangerines
- Tomatoes

## *Sauces and Dressings (with no added sugars)*

- Blue cheese
- French
- Italian
- Lemon juice
- Lime juice
- Salsa
- Ranch
- Soy
- Sugar free ketchup
- Vinegar
- Worcestershire sauce.

## *Spices & Herbs*

- Allspice
- Cajun
- Capers
- Chili powder
- Cinnamon
- Cream of tartar
- Cumin
- Dill
- Garlic powder
- Oregano
- Paprika
- Parsley
- Pumpkin spice

- Turmeric
- Pepper (has some carbs)

### *Fats & Oils*

- Béarnaise sauce
- Butter
- Bacon fat
- Coconut oil
- Duck fat
- Hollandaise sauce
- Mayonnaise
- Olive oil
- Peanut oil
- Sesame oil
- Sunflower oil

### *Other*

- Almond flour
- Chia seeds
- (Sugar free) cocoa powder
- Coconut flour
- Coconut flakes
- Flax meal
- Flax seeds
- Nuts
- Seeds

### *Sweeteners*

- Erythritol
- Stevia
- Xylitol
- Monk fruit powder

### *Liquids (without sugars)*

- Almond milk
- Cashew milk
- Coconut milk
- Coffee with heavy cream
- Teas and infusions
- Water - mineral water, flat or sparkling

### *Foods to avoid completely*

- Cakes
- Candy
- Chips

- Cookies
- Crackers
- Fruit juices
- Grains
- Honey
- Pasta
- Pastry
- Potatoes
- Rice
- Sugar
- Syrups
- Wheat breads

This list is incomplete and is to be used as a guide only.

Please note: If you are eating a ketogenic diet for **weight loss purposes**, it is necessary to avoid eating inflammatory foods. This includes all dairy products – milk, cheese, yogurt and so forth and all seed oils such as colza or sunflower. Instead, use nut butters and milks and olive or coconut oil.

# Chapter 5: Fat Bomb Recipes

Fat bombs are the perfect go to tool when you need something in between meals or as a handy breakfast or dessert. They are small, easy to prepare, satisfying and delicious, and can be either savory or sweet.

Fat bombs contain 3 types of ingredient:

- Healthy fats
- A flavoring
- Something to give them texture

Making them is super simple too, all you need is to:

- Add all the ingredients together
- Mix them up well
- Form them into balls using your hands, candy cups or spread out on a baking sheet then cut into squares
- Refrigerate until solid (several hours or overnight)

You can find 100's of fat bomb recipes on the Internet. Here are some of my favorite recipes to get you going. I hope you enjoy them.

### *Eggs and Bacon Breakfast Bombs*

Preparation 10 minutes Cooking Time 30 minutes
Makes 6 bombs

| | |
|---|---|
| Net carbs | 0.2 grams (0.007 ounces) |
| Fiber | 0 grams (0 ounces) |
| Protein | 5 grams (0.176 ounces |
| Fat | 18.4 grams (0.65 ounces) |

## <u>Ingredients</u>

- 4 large rashers of bacon
- 2 large eggs
- 1/4 cup softened butter
- 2 tablespoons mayonnaise (preferably homemade)

## <u>Method</u>

1. Pre-heat oven to 375 degrees Fahrenheit or 190 degrees centigrade
2. Line a baking tray with cooking parchment
3. Arrange the bacon rashers in rows with no overlap
4. Cook for 10 to 15 minutes until they are golden brown remove from oven and set aside to cool

5. Meanwhile, boil the eggs in a saucepan 2/3 filled with warm water. Allow to water to come to a gentle rolling boil slowly and boil for 10 minutes
6. Drain the eggs and fill the saucepan with cold water, once cool, peel the eggs in the water
7. Chop the eggs into quarters and add the warm butter, mash together then add the mayonnaise, salt and pepper. If there is any bacon grease in the pan after cooking the bacon add this too. Combine thoroughly.
8. Refrigerate the egg mixture for 30 minutes to harden
9. Once the bacon has cooled, chop it into small bits and spread it out on the baking sheet
10. Remove your egg mixture from the fridge and form it into approximately 6 equally sized balls (an ice cream scoop can be useful for this job)
11. Roll each ball in the bacon bits until evenly covered
12. Either eat straight away or keep refrigerated in an airtight container for up to 4 days

## *Pecan Nut and Maple Fudge Bombs*

Preparation 15 minutes Cooking and Cooling 1 to 2 hours

Makes 16 bombs

Net Carbs      1.4 grams (0.049 ounces)

Fiber          2.8 grams (0.098 ounces)

Protein        2.6 grams (0.091 ounces)

Fat            26 grams (0.917 ounces)

### <u>Ingredients</u>

- 3 cups of pecan nuts
- 1 teaspoon of vanilla extract
- ½ teaspoon ground cinnamon
- 1 teaspoon of sugar free maple extract
- Pinch of salt
- ¼ cup of Erythritol powder
- ½ cup of coconut oil
- 1 ¼ cups of chopped or halved pecan nuts

### <u>Method</u>

1. Place the 3 cups of pecan nuts, vanilla extract, cinnamon, maple extract and salt in a food processor and process until fully combined and smooth.
2. Add the erythritol powder and coconut oil and process until smooth.
3. Using a spatula, spread out on a baking sheet lined with baking parchment making sure it is even.
4. Decorate with the chopped or halved pecan nuts.
5. Refrigerate for several hours until solid.
6. Cut into 16 equally sized pieces and enjoy.
7. Can be kept in an airtight container in the refrigerator for up to one week.

## *Nutty Brownie Bombs*

Preparation 10 minutes Cooling 3 hours

Makes 24 Bombs

Net Carbs     2 grams (0.07 ounces)

Fiber     2 grams (0.07 ounces)

Protein     2 grams (0.07 ounces)

Fat     10 grams (0.35 ounces)

## <u>Ingredients</u>

- 1 cup of Coconut butter (warmed but not melted)
- ½ cup of Almond flour
- 4 tablespoons of Cocoa powder (unsweetened)
- 1 teaspoon of vanilla extract
- 3 tablespoons of coconut oil (gently melted)
- ¼ cup Brazil nuts (roughly chopped)

## <u>Method</u>

1. Place the coconut butter, almond flour, cocoa powder, vanilla extract and coconut oil into a bowl or food processor and mix until thoroughly combined.
2. Add ¾'s of the Brazil nuts and gently stir in.
3. Spread the mixture out onto a baking sheet lined with baking parchment.
4. Sprinkle the remaining Brazil nuts on top to decorate.
5. Refrigerate for 3 or more hours until solid.
6. Cut up into 24 equally sized bombs and enjoy.
7. Can be kept in an airtight container in the fridge for up to one week.

<u>*Breakfast*</u>

### *Creamy Strawberry Milkshake*

Preparation 5 minutes

Net Carbs    6.8 grams (0.24 ounces)

Fiber        2 grams (0.07 ounces)

Protein      2.5 grams (0.09 ounces)

Fat          27.4 grams (0.96 ounces)

Macronutrient ratio: Carbs 9.1%, protein 3.6%, Fat 87.4%.

## <u>Ingredients</u>

- ¼ cup of coconut milk (unsweetened)
- ¾ cup almond milk (unsweetened)
- ½ cup strawberries (hulked) can be fresh or frozen
- 1 tablespoon of MCT oil
- ½ teaspoon vanilla extract (sugar free)
- 1 tablespoon of chia seeds

## <u>Method</u>

1. Place all ingredients into a blender and pulse until smooth.
2. Serve immediately.

### *Ketogenic "All Day Breakfast"*

Preparation 15 minutes

Serves 1 portion

Net Carbs      6.6 grams (0.23 ounces)

Fiber          8.9 grams (0.31 ounces)

Protein        19.5 grams (0.67 ounces)

Fat            41.3 grams (1.45 ounces)

Macronutrient ratios: Carbs 6%, Protein 16%, Fat 78%.

## Ingredients

- 1 large free range or organic egg
- 5 bacon rashers
- 2 large mushrooms (Portobello).
- ½ Avocado (3.5 ounces)
- 1 tablespoon butter, virgin olive oil or coconut oil
- 1 teaspoon of garlic powder
- Freshly ground black pepper to taste
- Salt to taste
- Fresh chopped parsley as decoration if you want it

## Method

1. Place ½ of the butter or oil as you prefer into a non-stick frying pan and warm on a medium to low heat.
2. Add the mushrooms and garlic powder, salt and pepper and cook for about 5 to 8 minutes.
3. Remove mushrooms from the pan and keep them warm.
4. Rinse and dry the pan add the remaining butter or oil.
5. Fry the bacon on a medium heat until it is cooked the way you like it and remove it from the pan. Place with the mushrooms to keep warm.
6. Turn down the heat to low on the frying pan and crack in the egg, cook until it is the way you like it.
7. Halve an avocado and remove the stone.
8. Plate everything up and enjoy.

# <u>*Lunch*</u>

## ***Mexican Spice Bowl***

Preparation 20 minutes

Serves 4 servings

Net carbs       6.4 grams (0.22 ounces)

Fiber           3.7 grams (0.13 ounces)

Protein         17.6 grams (0.62 ounces)

Fat             31 grams (1.09 ounces)

Macronutrient ratios: Carbs 6.9%, protein 18.8%, fat 74.3%

## <u>Ingredients</u>

- 5 cups of Cauliflower "rice" (finely chopped cauliflower heart)
- 2 spicy chorizo sausages (8.5 ounces)
- 7 jalapeño peppers
- 3 tablespoons of freshly chopped parsley or cilantro if preferred
- 2 tablespoons of coconut oil (butter or lard can be used if not vegan)
- Salt to taste

## <u>Method</u>

1. Grate the head of the cauliflower to produce the "rice."
2. Slice up the chorizo into thin slices.
3. Chop and deseed the peppers.
4. In a greased skillet add the coconut oil or other fat and cook the peppers and chorizo until they are starting to brown, stir to prevent sticking.
5. Add the "rice" to the pan and cook for a further 8 to 10 minutes.
6. Season to taste (try before seasoning as some chorizo's have more salt added than others).
7. Plate up and scatter over the parsley or cilantro to decorate.

## *Salmon Stuffed Avocado*

Preparation 30 minutes

Serves 2

Net carbs        6.4 grams (0.22 ounces)

Fiber        7.5 grams (0.26 ounces)

Protein        27 grams (0.95 ounces)

Fat        34.6 grams (1.22 ounces)

Macronutrient ratios: Carbs 6%, protein 24%, fat 70%

## **Ingredients**

- 2 medium avocados with seed removed
- 2 small salmon fillets (7.8 ounces uncooked)
- 1 white onion chopped up finely
- ¼ cup of sour cream or mayonnaise
- 2 tablespoons freshly squeezed lemon juice
- Salt to taste
- Freshly ground black pepper to taste
- 1 tablespoon of coconut oil
- 1 tablespoon of fresh chopped dill
- 1 lemon cut into ¼'s as garnish

## **Method**

Heat the oven to 400 degrees Fahrenheit. Line a baking tray with baking parchment and place the salmon filets onto it. Drizzle the filets with 1 tablespoon of the lemon juice, a little olive oil, salt and pepper. Bake for 20 to 25 minutes.

Once cooked through remove the salmon from the oven and allow to cool for 10 minutes. Shred it using a fork but discard the skin. Add the chopped onion and mix it with the sour cream or mayonnaise and the dill.

Add the remaining lemon juice, salt and pepper and combine.

Scoop out the flesh of the avocado and cut into small cubes, add it to the fish mixture.

Place the mixture into the avocado shells and serve with the lemon wedges.

# *Dinner*

## *Pulled Pork with Pomegranate*

Preparation 15 minutes Cooking 7 hours or overnight

Serves 8

Net carbs       3.8 grams (0.13 ounces)

Fiber           1.4 grams (0.049 ounces)

Protein         35 grams (1.23 ounces)

Fat             36.6 grams (1.29 ounces)

Macronutrient ratios: Carbs 3.1%, protein 28.9%, fat 68%

## <u>Ingredients</u>

- 3 1/2 pounds of boneless pork shoulder joint
- 1 large white onion
- 1 fresh pomegranate
- 3 bay leaves
- 1 tablespoon of onion powder
- 1 tablespoon of garlic powder
- 1 tablespoon of paprika
- 1 teaspoon of smoked paprika
- 2 teaspoons of salt
- ½ teaspoon of freshly ground black pepper

## <u>Method</u>

1. Set slow cooker to high and allow to heat up.
2. Mix the onion powder, garlic powder, paprika, smoked paprika, salt and pepper in a bowl.
3. Score the pork skin with cuts 1 inch apart in both directions to make a diamond pattern.
4. Rub the spice mixture into the pork thoroughly.
5. Roughly slice the onion once peeled and put it into the slow cooker with the bay leaves.
6. Put the pork into the slow cooker on top of the other ingredients already there. Do not add any water.
7. Cook on high for approximately 5 to 6 hours or on low for around 8 to 10 hours (overnight). Exact time will depend on your slow cooker as they cook at different heats.
8. Once the pork is cooked take off the lid to remove the steam.
9. Preheat your oven to 400 degrees Fahrenheit and carefully remove the pork from the slow cooker and place on a baking sheet that has been lined with baking parchment.

10. Cook skin side up for 30 to 40 minutes to crisp the skin.
11. While the pork is in the oven remove the liquid and onions from the slow cooker and place into a blender (remove the bay leaves and discard). Pulse the blender to create a smooth sauce and set it to one side.
12. Cut the pomegranate in half and carefully remove the seeds placing them in a bowl.
13. Remove the port from the oven and using two forks pull the meat apart to shred it into small pieces.
14. Heat the sauce and pour it over the pork combining well.
15. Toss the pomegranate seeds through the pork and serve immediately.

### *Keto Vegan Curry Plate*

Preparation 25 minutes Cooking 45 minutes

Serves 6

Net carbs       10.7 grams (0.37 ounces)

Fiber             6.8 grams (0.24 ounces)

Protein           6.1 grams (0.21 ounces)

Fat               26.4 grams (0.93 ounces)

Macronutrient ratio: Carbs 14%, protein 8%, fat 78%

## <u>Ingredients</u>

- 2 tablespoons of virgin coconut oil
- 2 cups of vegetable stock
- ½ small white onion chopped
- 2 garlic cloves minced
- 1 teaspoon of ground cumin
- 1 teaspoon of ground coriander
- ½ teaspoon ground turmeric
- 1 teaspoon paprika
- 1 red chili pepper deseeded and diced
- 1 cup coconut milk
- 1 ¼ cups tinned tomatoes chopped
- 1 medium red bell pepper diced
- 1 medium zucchini cubed
- A large bunch of kale with stems removed then chopped
- 1 eggplant cut into cubes
- 3 tablespoons extra virgin olive oil
- ½ teaspoon of salt
- ¼ teaspoon of freshly ground black pepper
- 6 cups of cauliflower rice (cauliflower heart grated into rice like pieces)
- 4 tablespoons of coconut cream

## <u>Method</u>

1. In a pan simmer the stock on a medium to low heat for 15 minutes until the volume has been reduced by half.
2. Preheat the oven to 375 degrees Fahrenheit.

3. Put the eggplant chunks into a baking tray and drizzle them with olive oil and salt. Roast them for approximately 20 to 25 minutes until they are golden and soft.
4. Place the coconut oil into a clean saucepan and fry the onion on a medium heat until it becomes translucent. Add the chopped garlic and fry for another minute. Then add the bell pepper and zucchini and cook for 3 more minutes.
5. Add all the spices and stir well.
6. Next add the reduced stock, tomatoes and chili and season with the salt and pepper.
7. Simmer the pan on a low heat for 10 to 12 minutes before adding the coconut milk and simmering for a further 10 minutes.
8. Add the kale to the pot and allow it to wilt. Take the pan from the heat and add the rest of the olive oil and the eggplant. Combine thoroughly.
9. Plate up by serving the cauliflower rice with the curry. It can be garnished with more coconut cream if you wish and chopped cilantro.
10. The curry can be refrigerated in an airtight container for 5 days or frozen for 2 months.

* Please note that all measurements and values given in this book are meant as a guide and cannot be guaranteed to be 100% accurate.

# Conclusion

Look online to find 1000's of amazing ketogenic friendly recipes. You'll love the perfect way to get thin while eating amazingly filling and delicious food.

Don't forget to keep a food diary. It will help you to track your progress and highlight any problem areas. It isn't just for writing down what you eat each day but also how much weight you have lost each week and any other notes you find useful to keep.

Don't forget if you specifically want to lose weight, avoid all inflammatory foods, particularly dairy products and grain oils.

Ensure you only eat foods on the keto approved list and completely avoid all carbohydrate rich foods.

Remember it can take over a week for your body to get into a state of ketosis.

If you are unlucky enough to experience the symptoms of carbohydrate withdrawal, don't give up! Just tough it out and very soon you will be feeling great and by maintaining the diet you will lose weight.

Make sure that you check your macros carefully against what you eat every day. Keep a note in your food diary and ensure that you eat enough fat.

For extra speedy weight loss results you can try combining the Keto diet with intermittent fasting and exercise to benefit from a new you in no time flat.

I wish you a happy, healthy Keto journey.

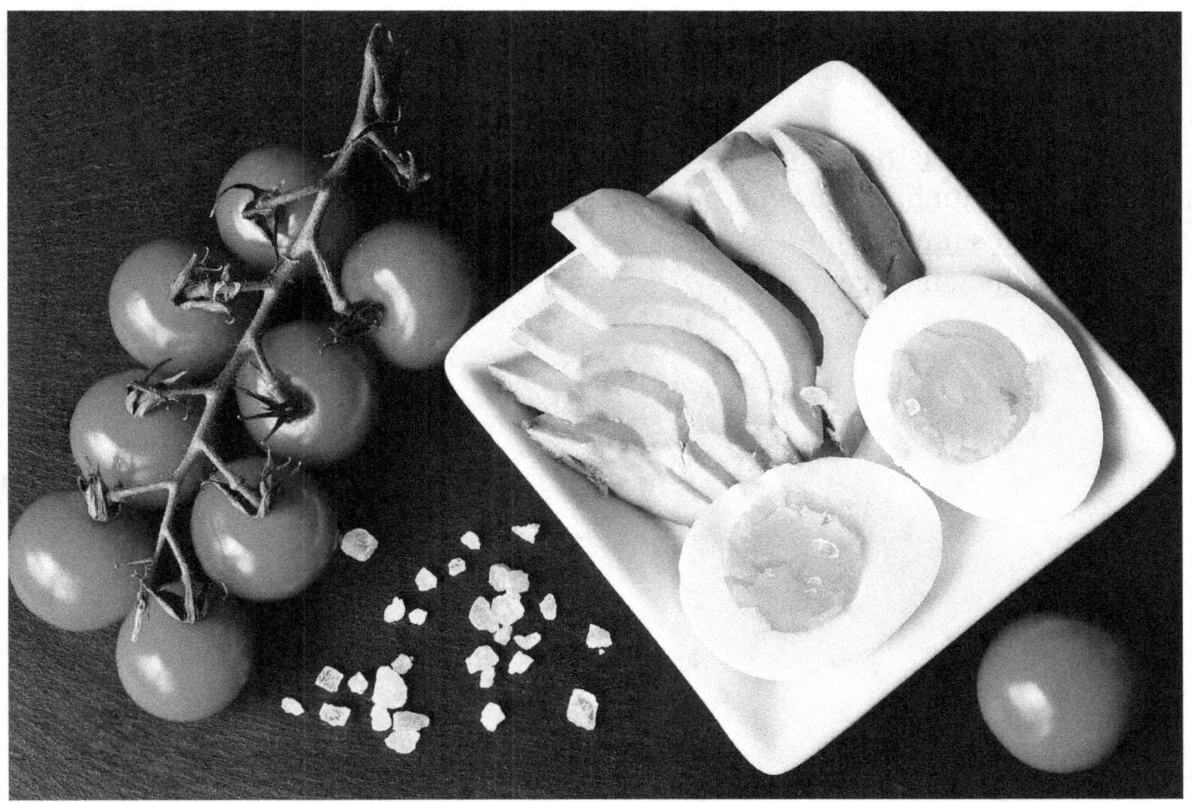

And finally, if you liked the book, I would like to ask you to do me a favor and leave a review for the book on Amazon. Just go to your account on Amazon or click on the link below.

**CLICK HERE TO LEAVE A REVIEW ON AMAZON!**

Thank you and good luck!

## References

https://ketobootstrap.com/recipe
https://ketosummit.com/what-are-keto-fat-bombs-recipes-how-to-make
https://ketosummit.com
https://ketodietapp.com